My Wonder Weeks
Diary

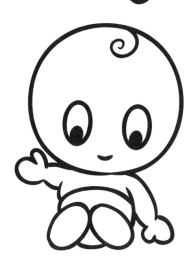

By Me and Xaviera Plas

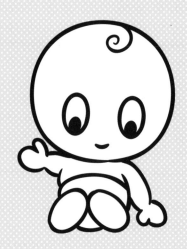

Congratulations!

You just made yourself the author of the best, most treasured book ever. This is a book that shows how your baby developed during the first year of his/her life.

Write as you and your baby experience each magical leap in this diary. The questions will help you to observe the typical traits of each Wonder Week. Don't know the answer to a question right away? Just take your time to look at this aspect of your baby's development before answering. You will see that this will become the best, most special book you will ever write.

Collect and create the best of each leap at the Scrapbook page. Be as creative as you want! Just stick all your special memorabilia on these pages. It might be a receipt of the latte you drank at that special little café where the waiters always compliment your baby, the label of the bear that was interesting to your baby this leap, or a lipstick kiss of grandma who, just like with every leap, kissed your baby all over. It's these little memories that make a big difference later on!

We would LOVE to see what you created! Please share your Scrapbook pages or any other pages with us! Mail them, post them, tweet them, or pin them! Have fun creating the best diary ever!

Love,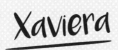

My Wonder Weeks Diary

Copyright © Kiddy World Publishing
Written by: Me & Xaviera Plas
Cover & Concept Creation by: Anita Peereboom
Illustrations by: Hetty van de Rijt, Vladimir Schmeisser
Layout by: Andrei Andras
Printed in Turkey

Kiddy World Publishing
Van Pallandtstraat 63
6814 GN Arnhem
The Netherlands

WWW.THEWONDERWEEKS.COM

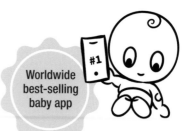

Worldwide
best-selling
baby app

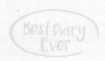

This diary belongs to:

your chart

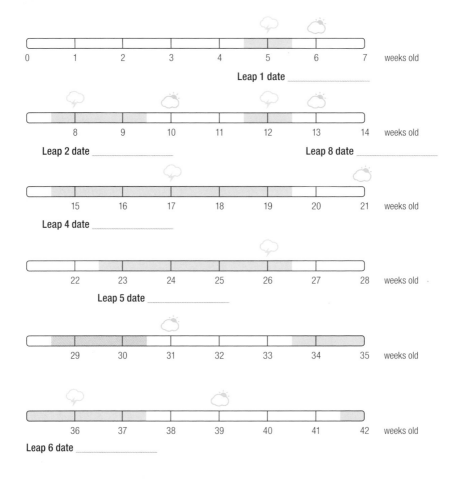

								weeks old
0	1	2	3	4	5	6	7	weeks old

Leap 1 date _____

| 8 | 9 | 10 | 11 | 12 | 13 | 14 | weeks old |

Leap 2 date _____   **Leap 8 date** _____

| 15 | 16 | 17 | 18 | 19 | 20 | 21 | weeks old |

Leap 4 date _____

| 22 | 23 | 24 | 25 | 26 | 27 | 28 | weeks old |

Leap 5 date _____

| 29 | 30 | 31 | 32 | 33 | 34 | 35 | weeks old |

| 36 | 37 | 38 | 39 | 40 | 41 | 42 | weeks old |

Leap 6 date _____

Wonder Weeks told me the date of birth is just for cakes, but mental development is calculated based on the due date.

I calculated your leaps by:

☐ Doing the math

☐ Checking The Wonder Weeks app

Date of birth: _____

Due date: _____

| | 43 | 44 | 45 | 46 | 47 | 48 | 49 | weeks old |

Leap 7 date _____

| | 50 | 51 | 52 | 53 | 54 | 55 | 56 | weeks old |

Leap 3 date _____

| | 57 | 58 | 59 | 60 | 61 | 62 | 63 | weeks old |

| | 64 | 65 | 66 | 67 | 68 | 69 | 70 | weeks old |

Leap 9 date _____

| | 71 | 72 | 73 | 74 | 75 | 76 | 77 | weeks old |

Leap 10 date _____

| | 78 | 79 | 80 | 81 | 82 | 83 | 84 | weeks old |

☐ Your baby is probably going through a comparatively uncomplicated phase.

☐ Fussy and irritable behavior at around 29 or 30 weeks is not a telltale sign of another leap. Your baby has simply discovered that this mommy can walk away and leave him behind. Funny as it may sound, this is progress. It is a new skill: He is learning about distances.

☐ Your baby may be more fussy now.

Around this week, a "stormy" period is most likely to occur.

Around this week, it is most likely that your baby's sunny side will shine through.

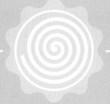

LEAP 1: THE WORLD OF

Changing sensations

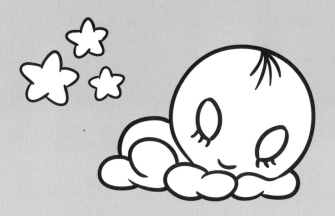

This wonder week's fussy signs

Date: _____

You are now making your first leap. I noticed this because you:

_____

_____

_____

On a scale of fussiness, I would say this leap is a:

1   2   3   4   5   6   7   8   9   10

The top three ways to soothe you were:

1. _____

2. _____

3. _____

This is how I felt:

_____

_____

_____

On a scale of feeling ☐ desperate / ☐ insecure / ☐ _____ I felt:

1   2   3   4   5   6   7   8   9   10

your three C's

The difference in:
Clinginess:

_____

_____

Crying:

_____

_____

Crankiness:

_____

_____

And don't forget about the difference in:
Sleeping:

_____

_____

Drinking:

_____

Although making a leap is not that easy, it's actually a sign that progress is on its way. The next pages will reveal what you have learned from the first leap you made.

Your emotions

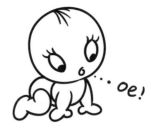

...oe!

I can see you show your emotions in a different way:

_____

_____

_____

_____

_____

Your smile:

_____

_____

_____

_____

_____

These are some physical changes that I noticed in regards to the little things like breathing, startling, trembling, crying, burping, and vomiting:

_____

_____

_____

_____

_____

your eyes

These are some pictures of things you like to look at. They are all simple little things, but they mean the world to you.

- ☐ You like to look and study the same things over and over again
- ☐ You get bored easily, and you want to see new things every time
- ☐ You look at objects longer and with more interest now
- ☐ The brighter the objects, the more interesting they are

your sounds & touches

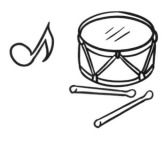

You react to sounds differently now than before in a way that:

_____
_____
_____

These sounds appeal to you most:

_____
_____
_____

These sounds scared you:

_____
_____
_____

The little noises you now make are:

_____
_____
_____

These are the ways you like to be touched now:

_____
_____
_____

your special activities

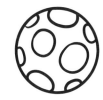

Everybody has their own personal activities they like to do with you!

These things you like to do most with:

_____
_____
_____

With _____ your most loved activities are:

_____
_____
_____

With _____ you like to:

_____
_____
_____

This is how you "tell" us you want a small break from all these activities:

- ☐ You look away for a moment
- ☐ You turn your head
- ☐ You close your eyes
- ☐ Your face shows me you're about to cry
- ☐ Other _____

your ten typicals

These ten things are so typically you:

1. _____

2. _____

3. _____

4. _____

5. _____

6. _____

7. _____

8. _____

9. _____

10. _____

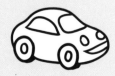

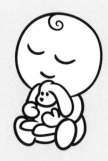

your firsts

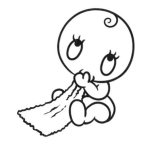

There's a first for everything, and during this leap, these were your firsts:

First

_____

_____

_____

First

_____

_____

_____

First

_____

_____

_____

First

_____

_____

_____

First

_____

_____

_____

your mighty milestones

My personal top 5 of all the developmental milestones you achieved are:

Milestone 1 _____

_____

_____

_____

Milestone 2 _____

_____

_____

_____

Milestone 3 _____

_____

_____

_____

Milestone 4 _____

_____

_____

_____

Milestone 5 _____

_____

_____

_____

Date of your first real social smile: _____

Date of your first real tear: _____

your special memory moments

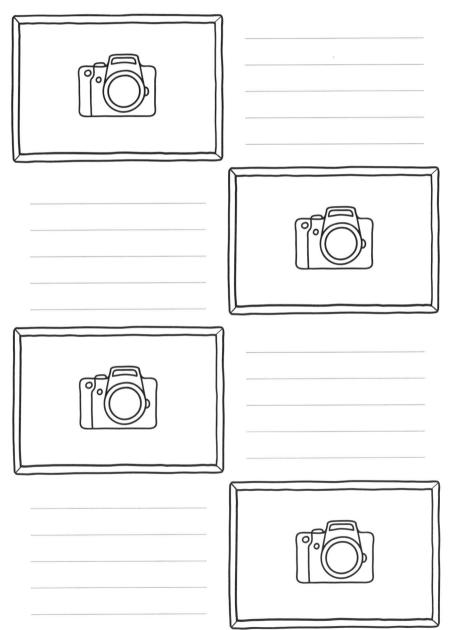

your first letter from me!

Congratulations!

Your leap is made!

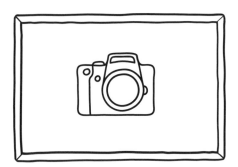

Your handprint:

Date: _____

Weight: _____

Height: _____

Size: _____

your leaply scrapbook

Cut out, stick, and keep all
your special memorabilia,
including receipts, tickets,
cards, drawings, little notes,
and photos!

The more, the better!
Collect and create
the best of each leap

My notes

LEAP 2: THE WORLD OF

Patterns

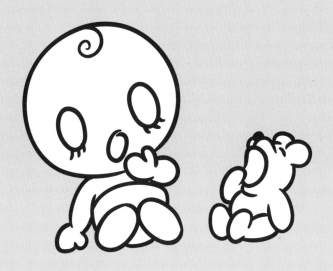

**YOUR BABY FEELS, HEARS AND SEES THEM…
FOR THE FIRST TIME**

This Wonder Week's fussy signs

Date: _____

You are now making your second leap. I noticed this because you:

_____
_____
_____

On a scale of fussiness, I would say this leap is a:

　　1　　2　　3　　4　　5　　6　　7　　8　　9　　10

The top three ways to soothe you were:

1._____

2._____

3._____

This is how I felt:

_____
_____
_____

On a scale of feeling ☐ desperate / ☐ insecure / ☐ _____ I felt:

　　1　　2　　3　　4　　5　　6　　7　　8　　9　　10

My cuddle care for you consists of:

_____
_____

your three C's

The difference in:
Clinginess:

_____

_____

Crying:

_____

_____

Crankiness:

_____

_____

And don't forget about the difference in:
Sleeping:

_____

_____

Drinking:

_____

_____

You...
- ☐ wanted more attention
- ☐ became shy with strangers
- ☐ clung to me more tightly
- ☐ slept poorly
- ☐ cried, cried, and cried some more

Yep, all this because progress is on its way. This leap made you perceive patterns for the first time in your life. The following pages are all about your exploration of the World of Patterns.

your body

You now move in another way:

_____

_____

_____

Your movements are a bit ☐ jerky/ ☐ rigid/ ☐ stiff/ ☐ like those of a puppet

These are the things you are now able to do with your body:

_____

_____

_____

With your hands you now:

_____

_____

_____

You looked very closely and saw _____

These are the body parts you now discovered:

_____

_____

_____

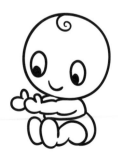

your love for visual patterns

Patterns are everywhere. Of all the patterns you saw around you, you love these the most:

your eyes

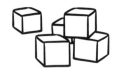

You now move and use your eyes in a different way:

_____
_____
_____
_____

When we go for a walk, you look at:

_____
_____
_____
_____

When you look at people, you like to look most at:

_____
_____
_____
_____

You now love to see...
- ☐ a flickering candle
- ☐ a waving curtain
- ☐ pets eating or moving
- ☐ people moving or eating
- ☐ bling, shiny clothing, or jewellery

your listening and chatting

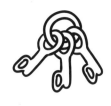

You react to sounds differently now than before in a way that:

_____

_____

_____

_____

_____

These are now the things you like to listen to:

_____

_____

_____

_____

_____

These sounds scared you:

_____

_____

_____

_____

_____

The short bursts of sounds you now are able to make sound like:

_____

_____

_____

_____

_____

your play

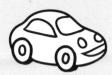

Your most beloved toys are now:

_____

_____

_____

_____

_____

These are the non-toy objects you like to "play" with or investigate at home:

_____

_____

_____

_____

_____

And these are the non-toy objects you like to "play" with or investigate outside our home:

_____

_____

_____

_____

_____

You prefer ☐ toys / ☐ "real things"

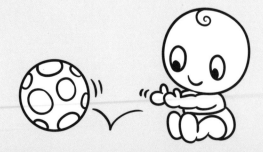

your special activities

Everybody has their own personal activities they like to do with you!

These things you like to do most with:

_____
_____
_____
_____
_____

With _____ your most loved activities are:

_____
_____
_____
_____
_____

With _____ you like to:

_____
_____
_____
_____
_____

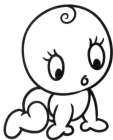

The World of Patterns

Your gymnastics, songs, & faces

These real body gymnastic games you like best now are:

_____

_____

_____

_____

The songs I sing for you are:

_____

_____

_____

_____

Faces! I love these different faces you make:

_____

_____

_____

_____

_____

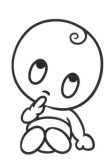

your first experiences

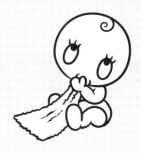

There's a first for everything, and during this leap, these were your firsts:

First
_____
_____
_____
_____

First
_____
_____
_____
_____

First
_____
_____
_____
_____

First
_____
_____
_____
_____

First
_____
_____
_____
_____

your special memory moments

...with pics to go along!

your typical yous

In our long chats, or better said my long monologues, I tell you:

_____

_____

_____

_____

The difference now, though, is that you start to "talk" back. I'm pretty sure you're telling me:

_____

_____

_____

_____

This is what I learned from you:

_____

_____

_____

_____

These words describe you and your character best now:

_____

_____

_____

_____

Most beautiful/ awesome/ humorous comment someone made about you:

_____

_____

_____

_____

your second letter from me!

Congratulations!

Your leap is made!

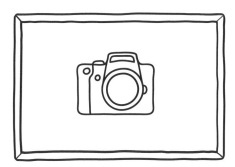

Your handprint:

Date: _____

Weight: _____

Height: _____

Size: _____

your leaply scrapbook

Cut out, stick, and keep all
your special memorabilia,
including receipts, tickets,
cards, drawings, little notes,
and photos!

The more, the better!
Collect and create
the best of each leap

My notes

LEAP 3: THE WORLD OF

Smooth Transitions

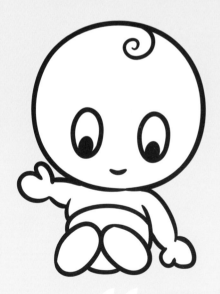

ONE THING CAN FLOW SMOOTHLY INTO THE NEXT

This Wonder Week's fussy signs

Date: _____

You are now making your third leap. I noticed this because you:

_____

_____

_____

On a scale of fussiness, I would say this leap is a:

☁ 1   2   3   4   5   6   7   8   9   10   ⛈

The top three ways to soothe you were:

1._____

2._____

3._____

This is how I felt:

_____

_____

_____

On a scale of feeling ☐ desperate / ☐ insecure / ☐ _____ I felt:

☁ 1   2   3   4   5   6   7   8   9   10   ⛈

Your three C's

The difference in:
Clinginess:

_____

_____

Crying:

_____

_____

Crankiness:

_____

_____

And don't forget about the difference in:
Sleeping:

_____

_____

Drinking:

_____

_____

You...
- ☐ became shy with strangers
- ☐ clung to me more tightly
- ☐ lost your appetite
- ☐ slept poorly
- ☐ sucked your thumb more often
- ☐ were listless

your body control

You seem to have a different type of body control than before the leap.
These are the main things I've noticed:

_____
_____
_____
_____

You move much more smoothly in this way:

_____
_____
_____
_____

The gymnastics and flexible tricks you perform with your body are:

_____
_____
_____
_____

Talking about "sitting," "rolling," and "holding" your head straight:

_____
_____
_____
_____

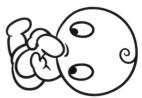

your hands & touches

Only a few weeks ago, you discovered these two things we call hands.

Already, you now:

_____

_____

_____

These are the things you like to do most with your hands:

_____

_____

_____

If you touch my face, you:

_____

_____

_____

If you touch your own face, you:

_____

_____

_____

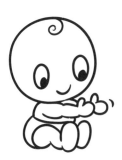

Your eyes

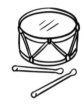

You can now follow something with your eyes in a smooth way.
This is a close-up picture of your eyes looking at your: _____

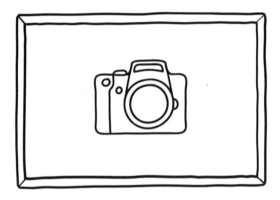

When you look at my face, you now look at:

_____
_____
_____
_____

You like to see the following smooth transitions around you:

☐ Lights being dimmed
☐ A hand going up
☐ A head being turned
☐ The smooth transitions in a toy
☐ Other _____

your emotions

You express your enjoyment through:

☐ Watching / Looking
☐ Listening
☐ Grabbing
☐ Talking then waiting for a response
☐ Other _____

You express different behaviour around different people. What I noticed:

_____

_____

_____

_____

_____

You show me you're bored by:

_____

_____

_____

_____

_____

Other new emotions I noticed were:

_____

_____

_____

_____

_____

your chats

You like to ☐ shriek / ☐ gurgle / ☐ make vowel-like sounds now all in a much smoother way than before the leap. These are the sounds you now make and when and where you do this:

_____
_____
_____
_____

If I imitate your sounds, you:

_____
_____
_____
_____

This is what I told you when we were chatting:

_____
_____
_____
_____

Your laugh tells my I've struck the right chord. This is what made you laugh this leap:

_____
_____
_____
_____

your play

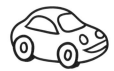

Your most beloved toys are now:

_____

_____

_____

These are the non-toy objects you like to "play" with or investigate at home:

_____

_____

_____

You started to explore the world by feeling all sorts of things:

_____

_____

_____

This is the music you like most now:

_____

_____

_____

I noticed this because this music makes you:

_____

_____

_____

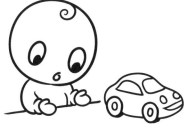

your firsts

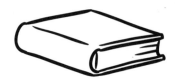

There's a first for everything, and during this leap, these were your firsts:

First
_____
_____
_____
_____

First
_____
_____
_____
_____

First
_____
_____
_____
_____

First
_____
_____
_____
_____

First
_____
_____
_____
_____

your mighty milestones

Milestone 1
_____
_____
_____
_____

Milestone 2
_____
_____
_____
_____

Milestone 3
_____
_____
_____
_____

Milestone 4
_____
_____
_____
_____

Milestone 5
_____
_____
_____

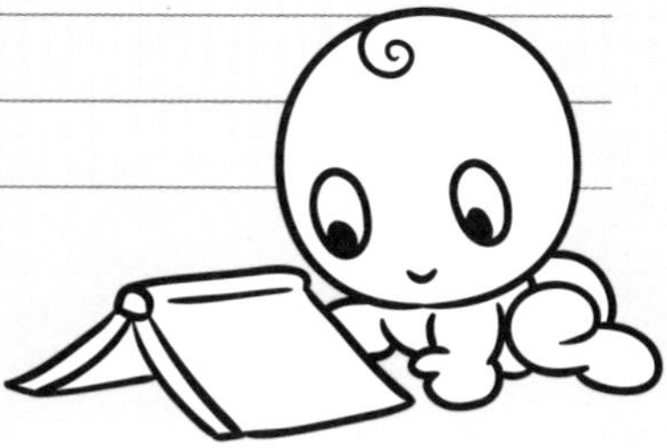

your special memory moments

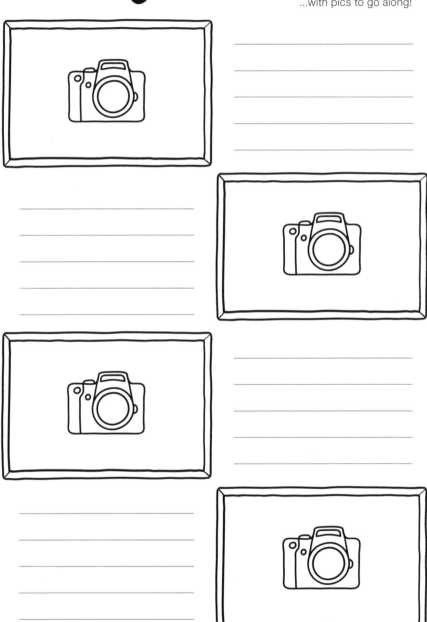

your typical yous

This is what I learned from you:

_____
_____
_____
_____

Looking back over a trimester of being together with you:

_____
_____
_____
_____

These words describe you and your character best now:

_____
_____
_____
_____

Most beautiful/ awesome/ humorous comment someone made about you:

_____
_____
_____
_____

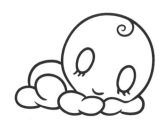

Your third letter from me!

Congratulations!

Your leap is made!

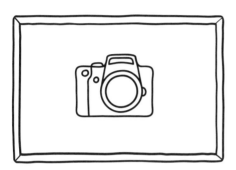

Your handprint:

Date: _____

Weight: _____

Height: _____

Size: _____

your leaply scrapbook

Cut out, stick, and keep all
your special memorabilia,
including receipts, tickets,
cards, drawings, little notes,
and photos!

The more, the better!
Collect and create
the best of each leap

My notes

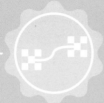

LEAP 4: THE WORLD OF

Events

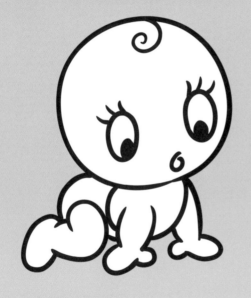

"

THE MOST TROUBLESOME LEAP OF ALL…

This Wonder Week's fussy signs

Date: _____

You are now making your fourth leap. I noticed this because you:

_____

_____

_____

On a scale of fussiness, I would say this leap is a:

    1   2   3   4   5   6   7   8   9   10

The top three ways to soothe you were:

1. _____

2. _____

3. _____

This is how I felt:

_____

_____

_____

On a scale of feeling ☐ desperate / ☐ insecure / ☐ _____ I felt:

    1   2   3   4   5   6   7   8   9   10

Your three C's

The difference in:
Clinginess:

_____

_____

Crying:

_____

_____

Crankiness:

_____

_____

And don't forget about the difference in:
Sleeping:

_____

_____

Drinking:

_____

You...
- ☐ had trouble sleeping
- ☐ became shy with strangers
- ☐ demanded more attention
- ☐ needed more head support
- ☐ wanted to always be with me
- ☐ lost your appetite
- ☐ were moody
- ☐ were listless

your exploration

It's clear that you perceive the world in a different way than before the leap. This is what I noticed:

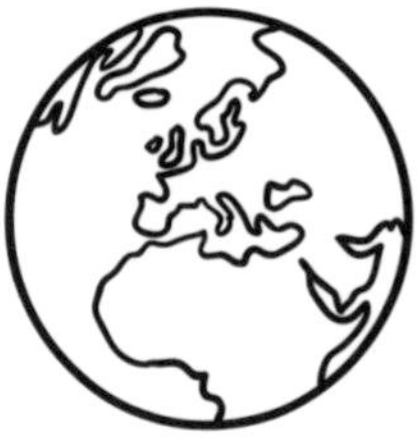

_____

_____

_____

_____

_____

_____

_____

_____

_____

_____

_____

_____

_____

_____

_____

_____

_____

_____

_____

_____

your way of examining

You are now able to make several flowing movements in succession.

As a result you...
- ☐ reach for
- ☐ grab
- ☐ pull

...toys towards you in one smooth movement to examine it.

You like to examine things by:
- ☐ Shaking
- ☐ Banging
- ☐ Poking
- ☐ Turning them around
- ☐ Sliding things up and down
- ☐ Putting the extra interesting things in your mouth

This is what and how you did this:

_____

_____

_____

_____

You feel with your mouth!
This is what you examined with your mouth:

_____

_____

_____

_____

your observations

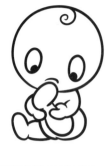

Sometimes you like to observe me doing things. For example:

_____
_____
_____
_____

Sometimes you body is too tired to continue the examination. I then help you by:

_____
_____
_____
_____

There are certain details of object that interest you to the max. These are:

_____
_____
_____
_____

Your most loved materials are:

_____
_____
_____
_____

your sight & seeing

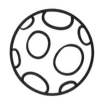

From all the daily chores, you like to watch:

_____

_____

_____

_____

Books… You're not reading them, but if I show you a colourful image on a page, you_____

If you look in the mirror or see me in the mirror, you:

_____

_____

_____

_____

These repetitive activities (i.e. jumping up and down, seeing someone brush his/her hair, or cutting bread) fascinate you most:

_____

_____

_____

_____

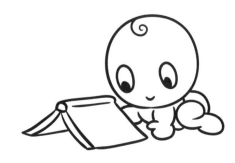

your chatting and listening

You are now able to make real babbling sentences. Lately you told me:

_____

_____

_____

You now experiment with intonations and volume:

_____

_____

_____

You are now able to make "events" with your voice using both your lips and tongue. These new sounds are:

- ☐ Ffft-ffft-ffft
- ☐ Vvvv
- ☐ Zzz
- ☐ Sss
- ☐ Brrrr
- ☐ Arrrr
- ☐ Rrrr
- ☐ Grrr
- ☐ Prrr

If you cough and I answer by "coughing back," you:

_____

_____

_____

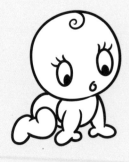

your body control & movements

These are the movement you now made and couldn't make before this leap:

_____

_____

_____

_____

You "ask" me to pick you by:

_____

_____

_____

_____

When I put you on the floor, you start to move:

_____

_____

_____

_____

You're now able to:

- ☐ Pass things from one hand to another
- ☐ Grab something if your hand comes in contact with it even without looking at it
- ☐ Grab things with either hand
- ☐ Shake a plaything
- ☐ Bang a plaything on a tabletop
- ☐ Deliberately throw things on the floor

your mouth & eating

When you had enough to eat, you:

_____

_____

_____

_____

If you see food or drinks or if you are hungry, you:

_____

_____

_____

_____

My mouth now seems really interesting to:

_____

_____

_____

_____

With your tongue, you now:

_____

_____

_____

_____

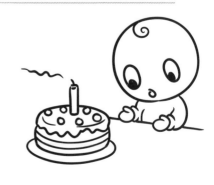

your special activities

Everybody has their own personal activities they like to do with you!

These things you like to do most with:

_____

_____

_____

_____

_____

With _____ your most loved activities are:

_____

_____

_____

_____

With _____ you like to:

_____

_____

_____

_____

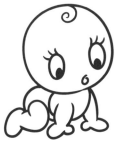

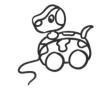

your firsts

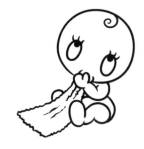

There's a first for everything, and during this leap, these were your firsts:

First
_____
_____
_____
_____

First
_____
_____
_____
_____

First
_____
_____
_____
_____

First
_____
_____
_____
_____

First
_____
_____
_____
_____

your mighty milestones

Milestone 1
_____
_____
_____
_____

Milestone 2
_____
_____
_____
_____

Milestone 3
_____
_____
_____
_____

Milestone 4
_____
_____
_____
_____

Milestone 5
_____
_____
_____
_____

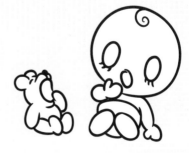

your special memory moments

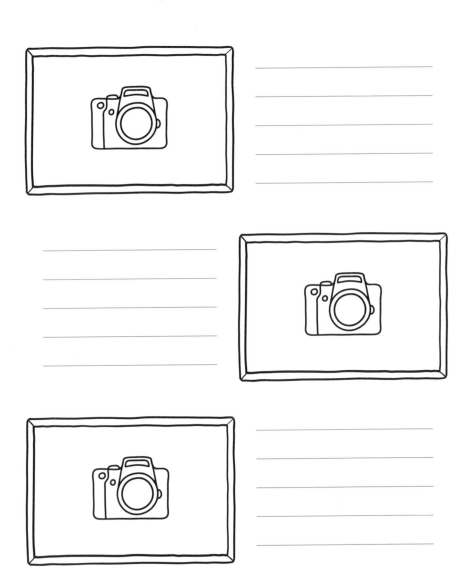

...with pics to go along!

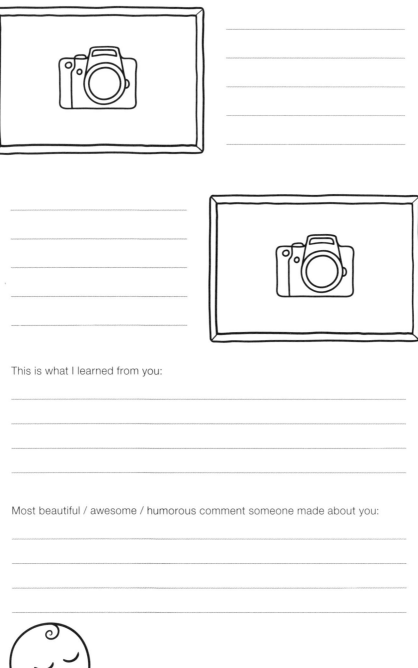

_____
_____
_____
_____

_____
_____
_____
_____
_____

This is what I learned from you:

_____
_____
_____
_____

Most beautiful / awesome / humorous comment someone made about you:

_____
_____
_____
_____

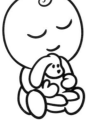

your fourth letter from me!

Congratulations!

Your leap is made!

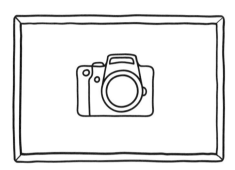

Your handprint:

Date: _____

Weight: _____

Height: _____

Size: _____

your leaply scrapbook

Cut out, stick, and keep all
your special memorabilia,
including receipts, tickets,
cards, drawings, little notes,
and photos!

The more, the better!
Collect and create
the best of each leap

My notes

Relationships

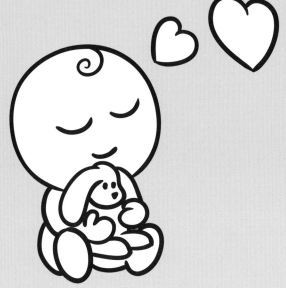

SEPARATION ANXIETY NOW REARS ITS HEAD

This Wonder Week's fussy signs

Date: _____

You are now making your fifth leap. I noticed this because you:

_____
_____
_____

On a scale of fussiness, I would say this leap is a:

☁   1   2   3   4   5   6   7   8   9   10   ☁

The top three ways to soothe you were:

1. _____
2. _____
3. _____

This is how I felt:

_____
_____
_____

On a scale of feeling ☐ desperate / ☐ insecure / ☐ _____ I felt:

☁   1   2   3   4   5   6   7   8   9   10   ☁

your three C's

The difference in:
Clinginess:

_____

_____

Crying:

_____

_____

Crankiness:

_____

_____

And don't forget about the difference in:
Sleeping:

_____

_____

Drinking:

_____

_____

LEAP 5

You...
- [ ] want me to keep you busy
- [ ] had "nightmares"
- [ ] lost your appetite
- [ ] are quieter and less vocal
- [ ] always wanted to be with me
- [ ] don't want me to change your diaper
- [ ] reached for cuddly objects more often
- [ ] were listless

your exploration

It's clear that you perceive the world in a different way than before the leap. This is what I noticed:

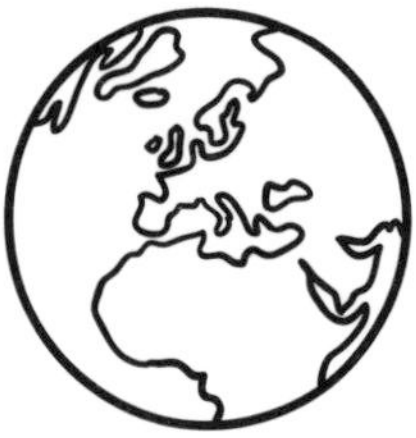

_____

_____

_____

_____

_____

_____

_____

_____

_____

_____

_____

_____

_____

_____

_____

_____

_____

_____

_____

your distance exploring

In, out, in front, behind, and next to are all keywords belonging to the leap of relationships. This is how I noticed you experimenting with these concepts:

_____

_____

_____

_____

The two things you like most to put in and out of each other are:

_____

_____

_____

_____

I've seen you studying the concept of distance by:

_____

_____

_____

_____

If I walk away and enlarge the distance between us, you:

_____

_____

_____

_____

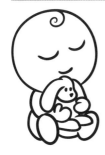

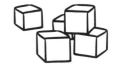

The World of Relationships

your actions result in

And you love experimenting with that.

You discovered these buttons and switches to flip:

_____

_____

You now realize things can be "taken apart," which is also a(n) (ex...) relationship between things. This is what you took apart:

_____

_____

You are tremendously interesed in examining little things like:
- ☐ Buttons
- ☐ Zippers
- ☐ Labels
- ☐ Stickers
- ☐ Marks on the wall
- ☐ Screws
- ☐ Other: _____

_____

This is a picture of you playing with a little detail:

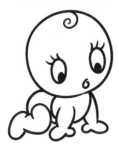

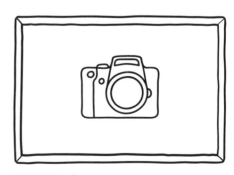

your body

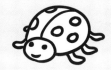

This is the way you now use your hands to grab:

_____
_____
_____
_____
_____

I've seen you lifting _____ to look under it. You saw:

_____
_____
_____
_____
_____

I've seen you mimicking these gestures:

_____
_____
_____
_____
_____

If you get your hands on a ball, you:

_____
_____
_____
_____
_____

your sight & seeing

When you observe adults, you like to look at:

_____

_____

_____

_____

The animal you like to watch most is:

_____

_____

_____

_____

I can see you looking from one thing to another:

_____

_____

_____

_____

_____

_____

_____

_____

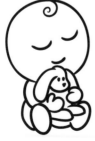 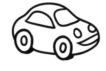

your smile

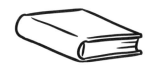

If somebody moves unusually, you:

_____

_____

_____

When I coincidentally let something fall on the ground, you:

_____

_____

_____

You laugh really hard when you see:

_____

_____

_____

_____

_____

_____

_____

_____

_____

_____

_____

_____

_____

your chatting and listening

When you hear music, your body:

_____
_____
_____
_____

You made the connections between the meaning of little sentences and the words! I can see you understand:

☐ No, don't do that

☐ Come on, let's go

☐ Others:

_____
_____
_____

When you hear voices or sounds coming out my phone, you:

_____
_____
_____
_____

You are trying to say words. Sometimes, I think I can almost make out that you are trying to say:

_____
_____
_____
_____

your first six months

You're my mini-me in the way that:

_____

_____

_____

_____

_____

_____

_____

_____

_____

_____

_____

_____

_____

_____

_____

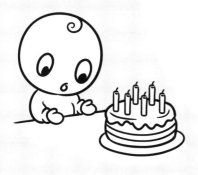

Your special activities

Everybody has their own personal activities they like to do with you!

These things you like to do most with:

_____

_____

_____

_____

_____

With _____ your most loved activities are:

_____

_____

_____

_____

_____

With _____ you like to:

_____

_____

_____

_____

_____

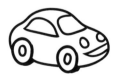

your mighty milestones

Milestone 1
_____
_____
_____
_____

Milestone 2
_____
_____
_____
_____

Milestone 3
_____
_____
_____
_____

Milestone 4
_____
_____
_____

Milestone 5
_____
_____
_____
_____

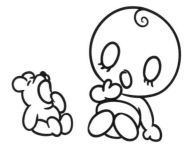

your special memory moments

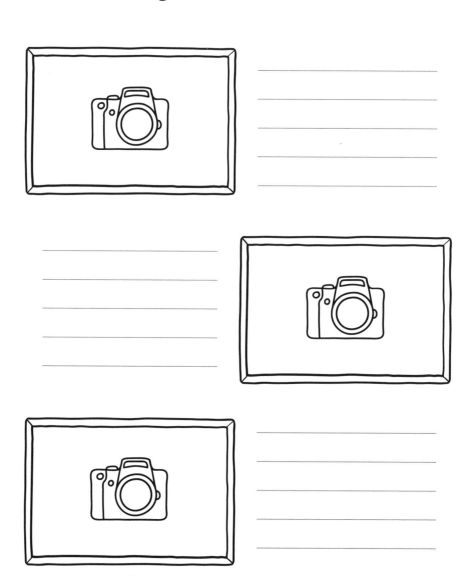

...with pics to go along!

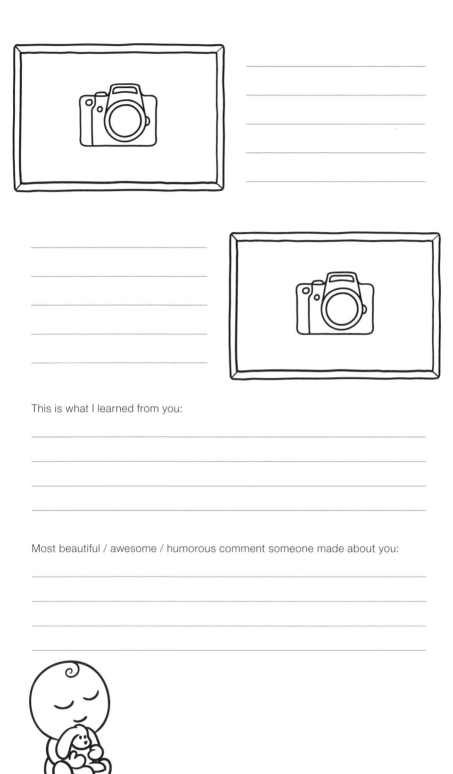

This is what I learned from you:

_____

_____

_____

_____

Most beautiful / awesome / humorous comment someone made about you:

_____

_____

_____

_____

your fifth letter from me!

Congratulations!

Your leap is made!

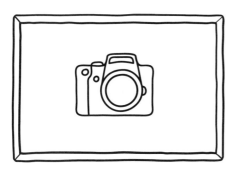

Your handprint:

LEAP 5

Date: _____

Weight: _____

Height: _____

Size: _____

your leaply scrapbook

Cut out, stick, and keep all
your special memorabilia,
including receipts, tickets,
cards, drawings, little notes,
and photos!

The more, the better!
Collect and create
the best of each leap

My notes

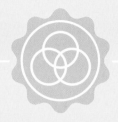

Categories

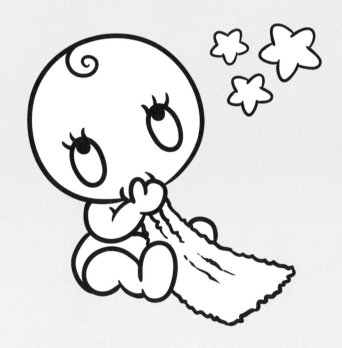

DIVIDING THE WORLD INTO GROUPS

This Wonder Week's fussy signs

Date: _____

You are now making your third leap. I noticed this because you:

_____
_____
_____

On a scale of fussiness, I would say this leap is a:

☁   1   2   3   4   5   6   7   8   9   10   ☁

The top three ways to soothe you were:

1._____
2._____
3._____

This is how I felt:

_____
_____
_____

On a scale of feeling ☐ desperate / ☐ insecure / ☐ _____ I felt:

☁   1   2   3   4   5   6   7   8   9   10   ☁

Your three C's

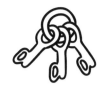

The difference in:
Clinginess:

_____

_____

Crying:

_____

_____

Crankiness:

_____

_____

And don't forget about the difference in:
Sleeping:

_____

_____

Drinking:

_____

_____

You...
- ☐ clung to my clothes
- ☐ were shy
- ☐ held on to me tightly
- ☐ demanded more attention
- ☐ had "nightmares"
- ☐ acted extra sweet
- ☐ were listless
- ☐ refused to get your diaper changed
- ☐ babbled less
- ☐ were less lively

Your recollection of

You showed that you could recognize a specific animal or person by:

_____

_____

_____

_____

_____

When I ask you where the _____ is in the book, you point it out!

You know when something is dirty. You show this by:

_____

_____

_____

_____

_____

You recognize and imitate expressions and movements of people:

_____

_____

_____

_____

_____

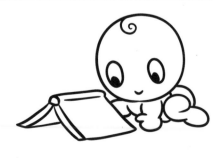

your emotions

When you look in the mirror, you:

_____
_____
_____
_____

If I pay attention to someone else, you:

_____
_____
_____
_____

When your teddy falls, you:

_____
_____
_____
_____

When you hear another child crying, you:

_____
_____
_____
_____

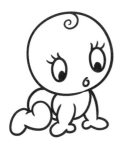

Your try-outs

You try to switch roles by:

- ☐ Playing peek-a-boo with a younger baby
- ☐ Feeding the bottle to me
- ☐ Inviting me to sing a song and then start clapping your hands
- ☐ Handing me the blocks to build a tower
- ☐ Other _____

This is a story about the first time you showed me you wanted to switch roles:

_____

_____

_____

_____

_____

_____

_____

_____

_____

_____

_____

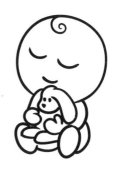

your exploring by investigation

Categories are groups of things with the same characteristics. And you already start to explore these categories and characteristics now.

Categories you were investigating with your toys:

_____

_____

_____

Categories you were investigating in humans:

_____

_____

_____

Categories you were investigating in our house:

_____

_____

_____

You explored categories like stickiness/ roughness / warmth / slipperiness by:

_____

_____

_____

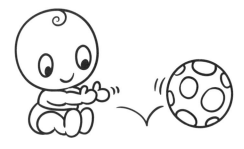

your chatting & laughing

You have a different sound-word for everybody in our family.

Here's how you call everybody:

_____
_____
_____
_____
_____
_____

The words I'm sure you now really understand are:

_____
_____
_____
_____
_____
_____

What made you laugh most was:

_____
_____
_____
_____
_____
_____

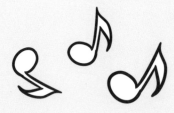

Your examinations

Inside, you love to examine:

_____

_____

_____

_____

Outside, you love to examine:

_____

_____

_____

_____

With _____ you like to examine:

_____

_____

_____

_____

In terms of demolition, you like to examine:

_____

_____

_____

_____

your special activities

These things you like to do most with:

_____

_____

_____

_____

_____

With _____ your most loved activities are:

_____

_____

_____

_____

_____

With _____ you like to:

_____

_____

_____

_____

_____

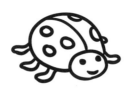

your mighty milestones

Milestone 1
_____
_____
_____
_____

Milestone 2
_____
_____
_____
_____

Milestone 3
_____
_____
_____
_____

Milestone 4
_____
_____
_____
_____

Milestone 5
_____
_____
_____

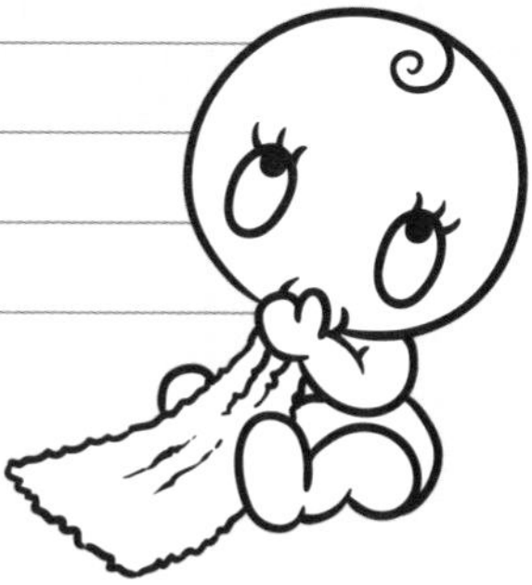

your special memory moments

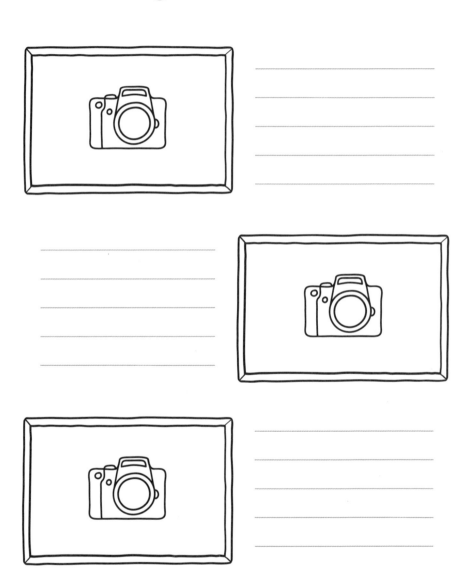

...with pics to go along!

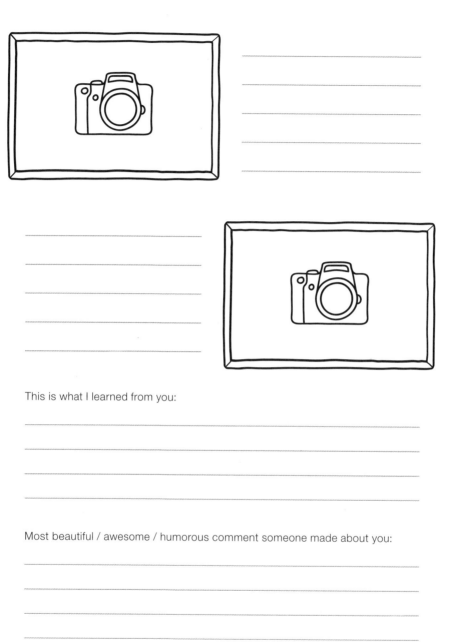

This is what I learned from you:

_____

_____

_____

_____

Most beautiful / awesome / humorous comment someone made about you:

_____

_____

_____

_____

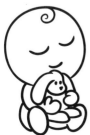

your sixth letter from me!

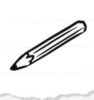

Congratulations!

Your leap is made!

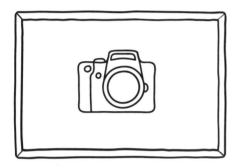

Your handprint:

Date:

Weight:

Height:

Size:

your leaply scrapbook

Cut out, stick, and keep all
your special memorabilia,
including receipts, tickets,
cards, drawings, little notes,
and photos!

The more, the better!
Collect and create
the best of each leap

My notes

Sequences

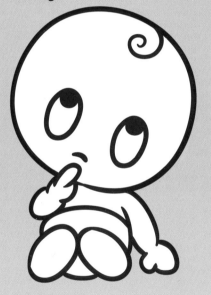

DOING TWO THINGS CONSECUTIVELY

This Wonder Week's fussy signs

Date: _____

You are now making your fourth leap. I noticed this because you:

_____

_____

_____

On a scale of fussiness, I would say this leap is a:

1   2   3   4   5   6   7   8   9   10

The top three ways to soothe you were:

1. _____

2. _____

3. _____

This is how I felt:

_____

_____

_____

On a scale of feeling ☐ desperate / ☐ insecure / ☐ _____ I felt:

1   2   3   4   5   6   7   8   9   10

My cuddle care for you consists of:

_____

_____

Your three C's

The difference in:
Clinginess:

_____

_____

Crying:

_____

_____

Crankiness:

_____

_____

And don't forget about the difference in:
Sleeping:

_____

_____

Drinking:

_____

You...
- [ ] were shy with others
- [ ] wanted to be kept busy
- [ ] were jealous
- [ ] were listless
- [ ] refused to get your diaper changed
- [ ] lost you appetite
- [ ] behaved more babyish
- [ ] acted unusually sweet
- [ ] were cheerful one moment, crying the next
- [ ] babbled less
- [ ] sat there, quietly dreaming
- [ ] sucked your thumb more often
- [ ] cuddled toys more often

your pointing & talking

You try to get me to tell you the names of objects, people, and animals by:

_____
_____
_____

When I say someone's name and that person is around, you:

_____
_____
_____

If I ask you where your _____ is, you:

_____
_____
_____

These are the animals sounds you make when I ask you what this animals says:

_____
_____
_____

These are the words or sounds you make now:

_____
_____
_____

your doings

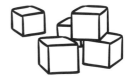

If I give you a key, you:

_____

_____

_____

_____

If I switch on the light, you:

_____

_____

_____

_____

If I put you in the sandpit with a small shovel, you:

_____

_____

_____

_____

If I give you blocks, you:

_____

_____

_____

_____

your tool-using, goal-reaching skills

When you try to get up or "walk" around, you:

_____
_____
_____
_____
_____

If you can't reach something, you:

_____
_____
_____
_____
_____

When you want me to take you in a specific direction, you:

_____
_____
_____
_____
_____

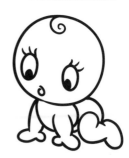

Your sequences

These are some example sequences you now did:

First you   Then you

_____   _____
_____   _____
_____   _____
_____   _____
_____   _____
_____   _____
_____   _____
_____   _____
_____   _____
_____   _____
_____   _____
_____   _____
_____   _____
_____   _____
_____   _____
_____   _____
_____   _____

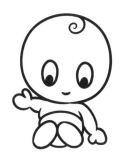

Your construction

The first thing you constructed was:

_____

_____

_____

_____

_____

The first time I saw you putting things together was:

_____

_____

_____

_____

I see you are linking things:

_____

_____

_____

_____

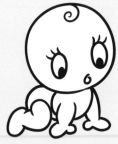

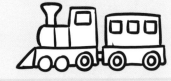

your eating

These are the funny things you do when you eat:

_____

_____

_____

_____

_____

You seem to want to share your food with:

_____

_____

_____

_____

_____

You want ☐ me to feed you / ☐ to feed yourself.

If I give you a spoon and your food, you:

_____

_____

_____

_____

_____

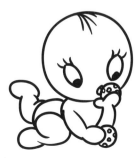

Your special activities

Everybody has their own personal activities they like to do with you!

These things you like to do most with:

_____

_____

_____

_____

_____

With _____ your most loved activities are:

_____

_____

_____

_____

_____

With _____ you like to

_____

_____

_____

_____

_____

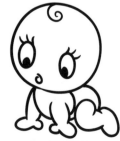

your games & toys

(& household things you see as toys)

Your most loved nursery rhyme: _____

When you hear it, you:

_____
_____
_____
_____

Your most loved toys are now:

_____
_____
_____
_____

After spending almost a year with you, I think these kinds of things appeal most to your character:

_____
_____
_____
_____

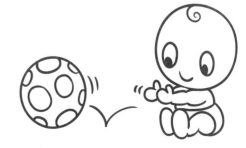

your firsts

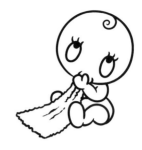

There's a first for everything, and during this leap, these were your firsts:

First
_____

_____

_____

_____

First
_____

_____

_____

_____

First
_____

_____

_____

_____

First
_____

_____

_____

_____

First
_____

_____

_____

_____

your mighty milestones

Milestone 1

_____
_____
_____
_____

Milestone 2

_____
_____
_____
_____

Milestone 3

_____
_____
_____
_____

Milestone 4

_____
_____
_____
_____

Milestone 5

_____
_____
_____
_____

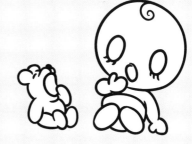

The World of Sequences

Your special memory moments

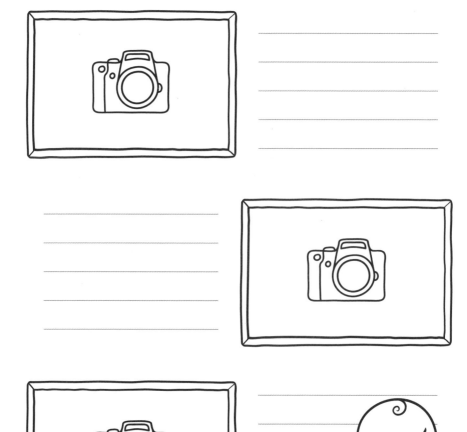

...with pics to go along!

your seventh letter from me!

Congratulations!

Your leap is made!

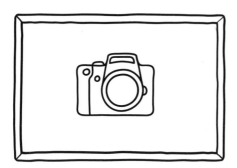

Your handprint:

Date: _____

Weight: _____

Height: _____

Size: _____

your leaply scrapbook

Cut out, stick, and keep all
your special memorabilia,
including receipts, tickets,
cards, drawings, little notes,
and photos!

The more, the better!
Collect and create
the best of each leap

My notes

One Year

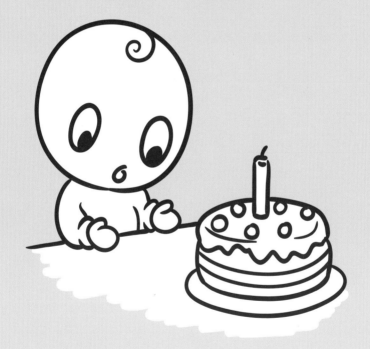

HAPPY FIRST BIRTHDAY!

One year

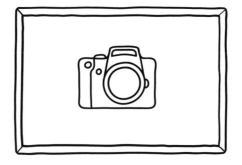

_____

_____

_____

These people came to congratulate you on your very first birthday:

_____

_____

_____

_____

_____

These are the presents that you received:

_____

_____

_____

_____

_____

This is what you did on your day in the spotlight:

_____

_____

_____

_____

_____

Happy First Birthday!

My notes

"The Wonder Weeks series

The Wonder Weeks is a #1 worldwide bestseller and a multi-award winning book!

✓ Gives insight in baby's 10 major mental developmental leaps

✓ Explains the fussy phases every child experiences

✓ Shows when new skills can appear

✓ Gives parents tools to help their baby through the fussy phases

✓ Offers parents support

➕ **EXTRA:** Insights, Tips & Tricks for Sleep & Leaps

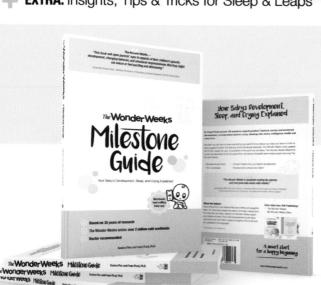

Your baby's Development, Sleep and Crying Explained

The Wonder Weeks Milestone Guide

The Milestone Guide provides information on other topics than those related to mental health as they are explained in The Wonder Weeks. Used together with The Wonder Weeks, they are the most complete resources for you to turn to.

But there's more!

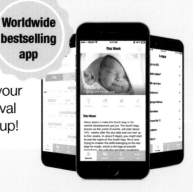

The Wonder Weeks App

Find out all about the leaps, at your fingertips, on your phone. **The #1 bestselling app,** the ultimate survival guide. Let us text you when a new leap is coming up!

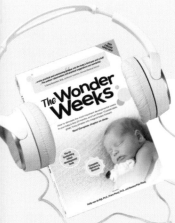

The Wonder Weeks Audio Book

Always on the run or do you just prefer to listen to a book? Download our audio app book. You can find it in the Apple App store or Google Play store.

The Wonder Weeks Online Guide

If you want to dive into the perceptual world of your baby… let us take you on a journey with movies, sounds, visuals and much more…

www.thewonderweeksonlineguide.com

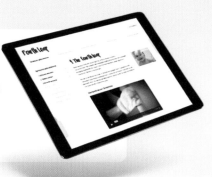

A true Wonder Weeks experience!

www.thewonderweeks.com